I0830102

endorsement or affiliation unless used under fair use principles or with proper permissions and attributions.

For permissions, inquiries, or requests regarding the book's use, please contact BINISH SHAH through official channels listed on their Amazon author page or provided email address.

This comprehensive copyright notice serves to protect BINISH SHAH's intellectual property rights, maintain content control, and inform users about associated restrictions and permissions.

Warm regards,

BINISH SHAH

The Amazing Apple
A Fun Guide to the
Benefits of Apples

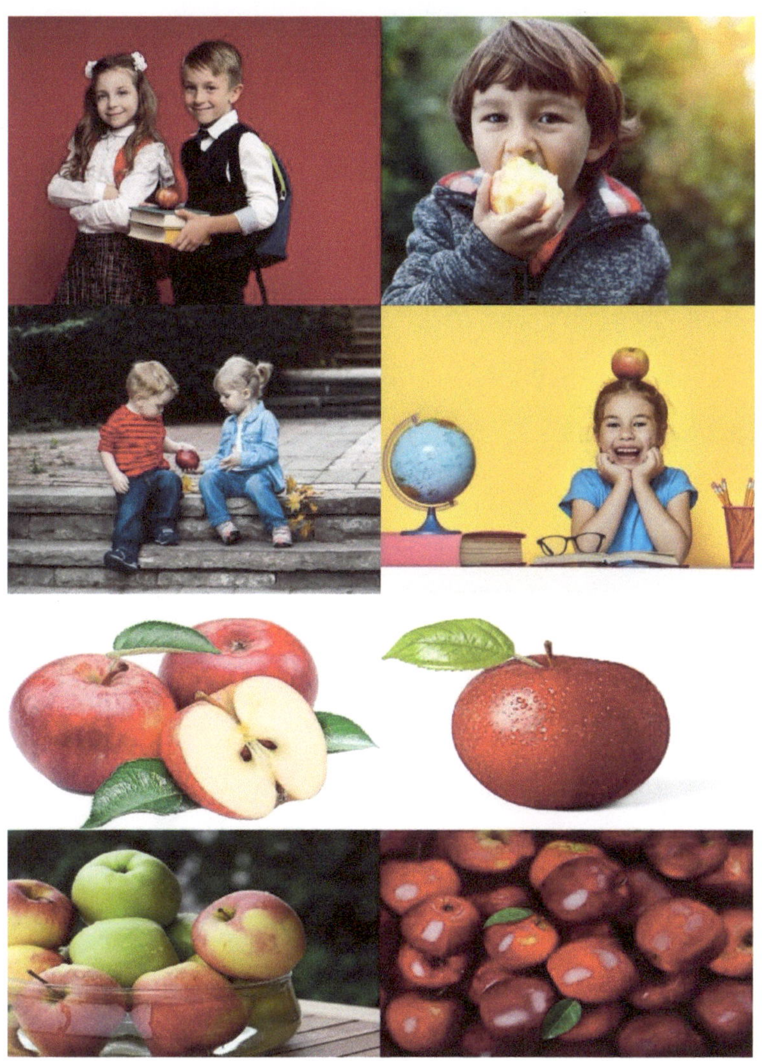

Table of Content

Preface

Welcome to "The Amazing Apple: A Fun Guide to the Benefits of Apples"! In this book, we invite you to embark on a delicious and educational journey into the world of apples.

Apples are not just tasty fruits – they're also packed with nutrients that are good for your body and mind. From vitamins and minerals to antioxidants and fiber, apples offer a wide range of health benefits that can help you grow strong, stay healthy, and feel happy.

Through colorful illustrations and easy-to-understand explanations, this book will show you just how amazing apples can be. You'll learn how apples can boost your immune system, keep your heart healthy, improve your digestion, and even enhance your mood.

Whether you're a fan of sweet Red Delicious apples or tart Granny Smiths, there's no denying that apples are a super food that can benefit everyone. So, grab a juicy apple, turn the page, and discover all the wonderful ways that apples can benefit your health and well-being.

Chapter 1: An Apple a Day Keeps the Doctor Away

Have you ever heard the saying, "An apple a day keeps the doctor away"? It turns out, there's a lot of truth to that! Apples are not only delicious but also incredibly good for you. In this chapter, we'll explore how eating apples can help keep you healthy and strong.

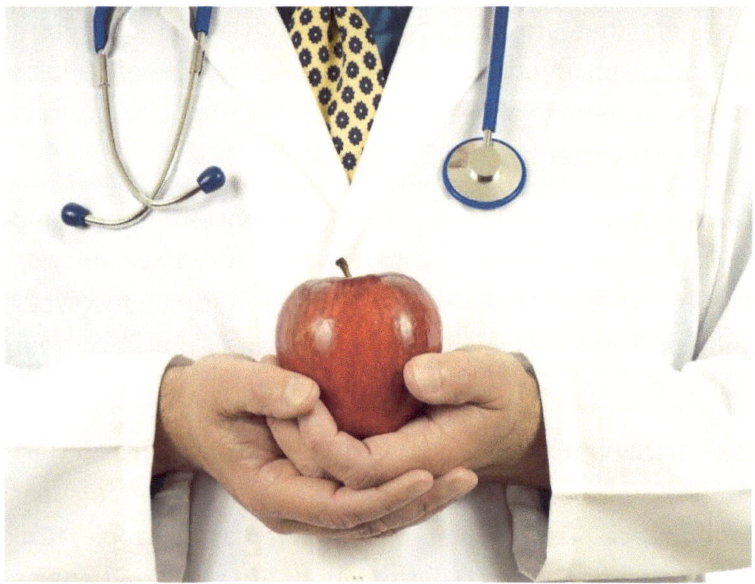

Apples are packed with vitamins and minerals that are essential for your body. One of the key vitamins in apples is vitamin C, which is known for its immune-boosting properties. Vitamin C helps your body fight off illnesses and keeps your immune system strong. So, by eating apples, you're giving your body a natural defense against colds, flu, and other infections.

But that's not all – apples are also rich in other vitamins and minerals, like vitamin A, vitamin K, and potassium. Vitamin A is important for maintaining good vision and healthy skin, while vitamin K is essential for blood clotting and bone health. Potassium, on the other hand, helps regulate your blood pressure and keeps your heart healthy.

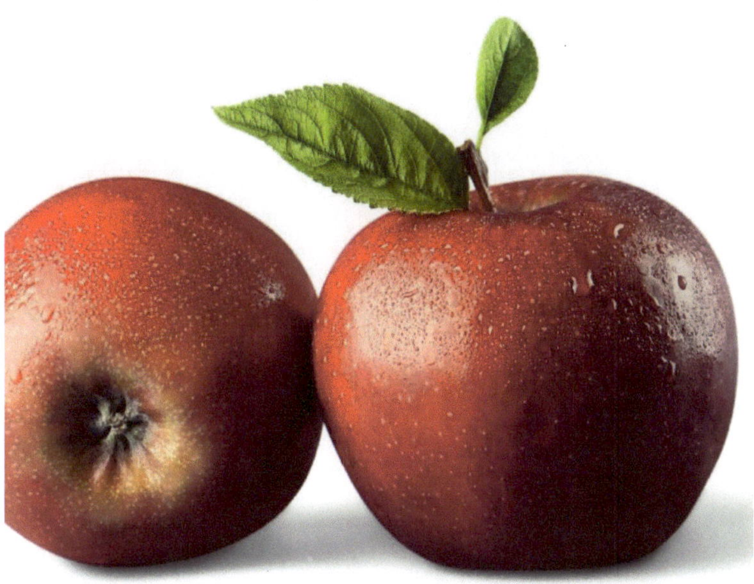

In addition to vitamins and minerals, apples are also a great source of fiber. Fiber is important for your digestive system, helping to keep things running smoothly and preventing constipation. It also helps you feel full, which can be helpful if you're trying to maintain a healthy weight.

So, the next time you're looking for a snack, reach for an apple! Not only are they delicious, but they're also packed with vitamins, minerals, and fiber that can help keep you healthy and strong.

Chapter 2: Grow Strong with Apples

Do you want to grow big and strong? Apples can help! In this chapter, we'll explore how the nutrients in apples can support your growth and help you develop healthy bones and muscles.

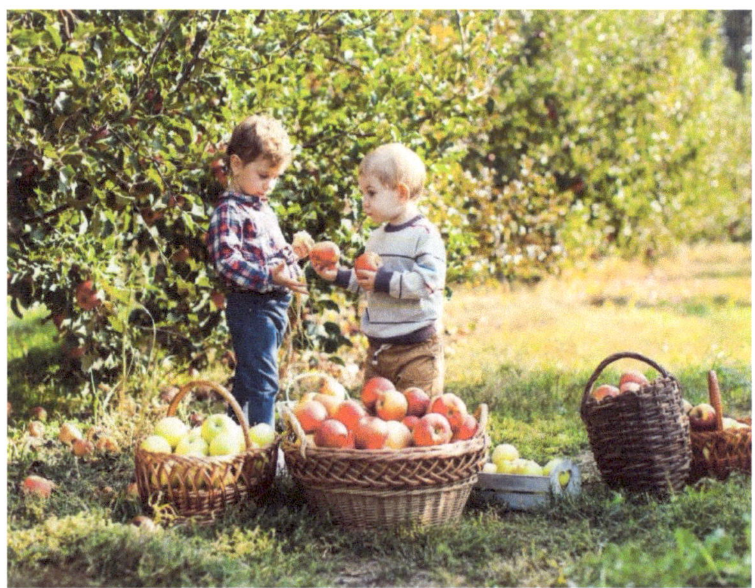

Apples contain several nutrients that are essential for bone health. One of these nutrients is calcium, which is crucial for building strong bones and teeth. Calcium also plays a role in muscle function and nerve signaling, making it essential for overall health.

Another important nutrient in apples is vitamin K, which is necessary for bone metabolism and the formation of bone tissue. Vitamin K helps regulate calcium in the body and ensures that it is deposited in the bones, where it is needed for strength and structure.

In addition to calcium and vitamin K, apples also contain magnesium, which is important for bone health. Magnesium helps regulate calcium levels in the body and is involved in the formation of bone tissue. It also plays a role in muscle function and energy production, making it essential for overall growth and development.

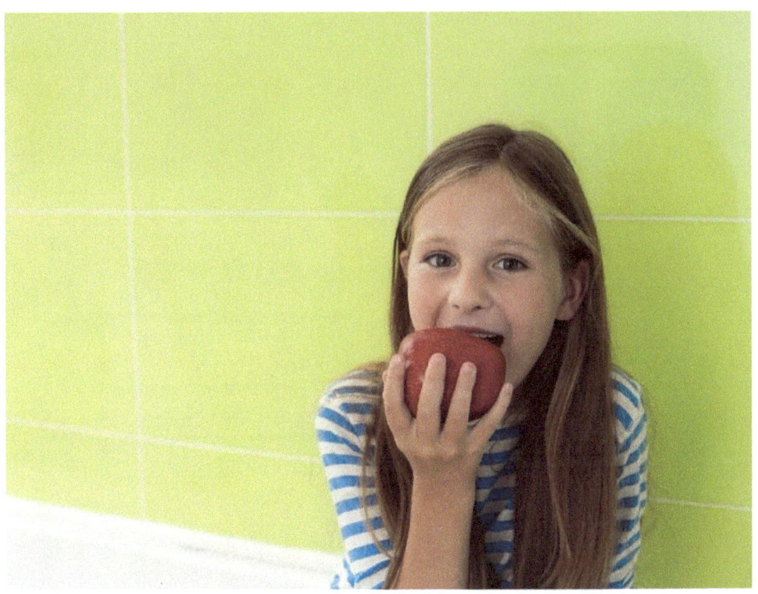

So, by eating apples, you're not only getting a delicious snack but also providing your body with the nutrients it needs to grow big and strong. Incorporating apples into your diet can help support healthy bones and muscles, ensuring that you reach your full potential.

Chapter 3: An Apple for Your Brain

Did you know that apples can help keep your brain sharp and focused? In this chapter, we'll explore how the antioxidants in apples can protect your brain cells and improve your memory.

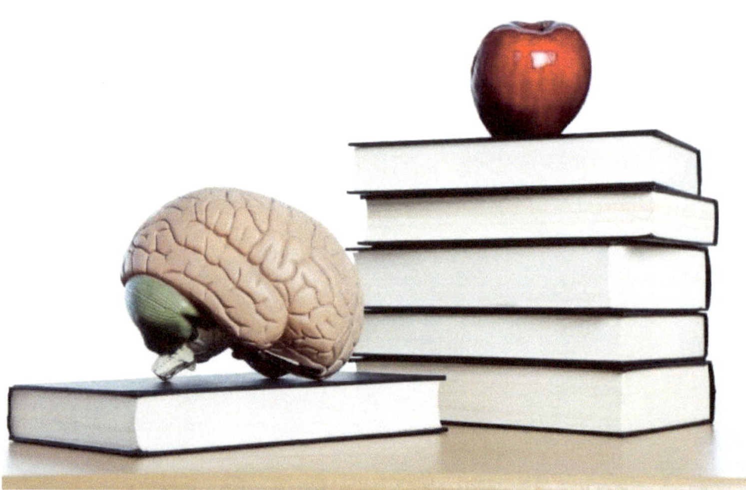

Apples contain antioxidants, such as quercetin and catechin, which have been shown to have neuroprotective effects. These antioxidants help protect your brain cells from oxidative stress, which can damage cells and lead to cognitive decline.

Oxidative stress is thought to play a role in the development of neurodegenerative diseases, such as Alzheimer's and Parkinson's disease. By eating apples, you can help reduce the risk of these diseases and keep your brain healthy.

In addition to protecting your brain cells, the antioxidants in apples can also improve your memory. Studies have shown that quercetin, in particular, may enhance memory and learning ability by promoting the growth of new brain cells and improving communication between brain cells.

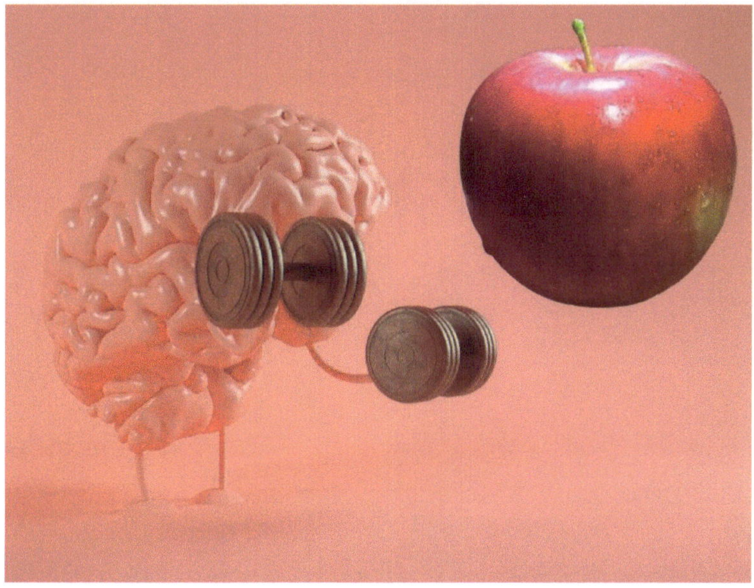

So, next time you're studying for a test or need to stay focused, reach for an apple! Not only will it provide you with a delicious snack, but it will also help keep your brain sharp and focused.

Chapter 4: An Apple for Your Heart

Your heart works hard every day to keep you alive, so it's important to take care of it. In this chapter, we'll explore how apples can keep your heart healthy and happy.

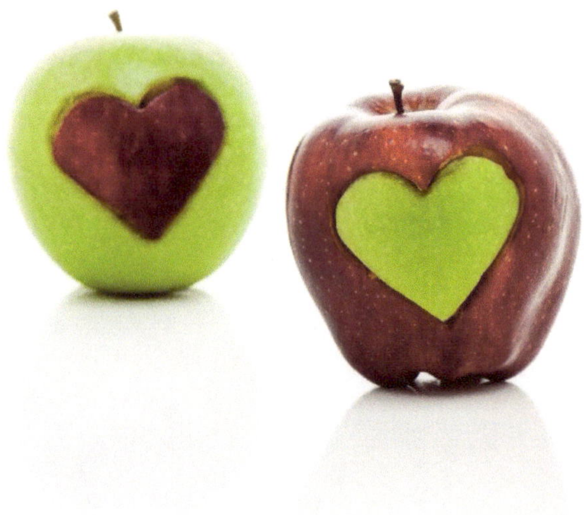

Apples are rich in fiber, which is good news for your heart. Fiber helps lower cholesterol levels, specifically the "bad" LDL cholesterol that can clog your arteries and lead to heart disease. By eating apples, you can help reduce your risk of heart disease and keep your heart pumping strong.

In addition to fiber, apples also contain antioxidants, such as flavonoids and polyphenols, which have been linked to a reduced risk of heart disease. These antioxidants help reduce inflammation in the body and prevent damage to your blood vessels, keeping your heart healthy and your blood flowing smoothly.

Studies have shown that eating apples regularly can lower the risk of heart disease and stroke. So, by adding apples to your diet, you're not only enjoying a tasty snack but also taking a big step towards keeping your heart healthy and happy.

Next time you're craving a snack, reach for an apple and give your heart some love!

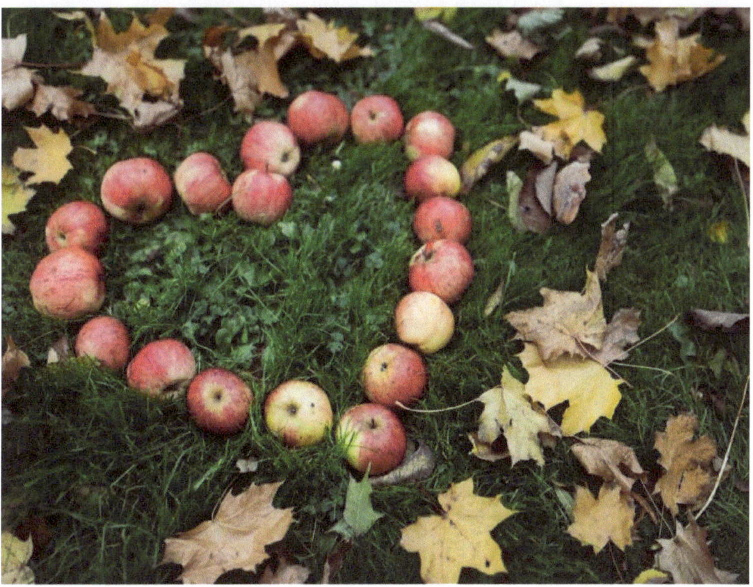

Chapter 5: An Apple for Your Tummy

Your tummy, or digestive system, plays a crucial role in your overall health. Luckily, apples can help keep your tummy happy and aid digestion. In this chapter, we'll explore how the fiber in apples promotes a healthy digestive system and prevents tummy troubles.

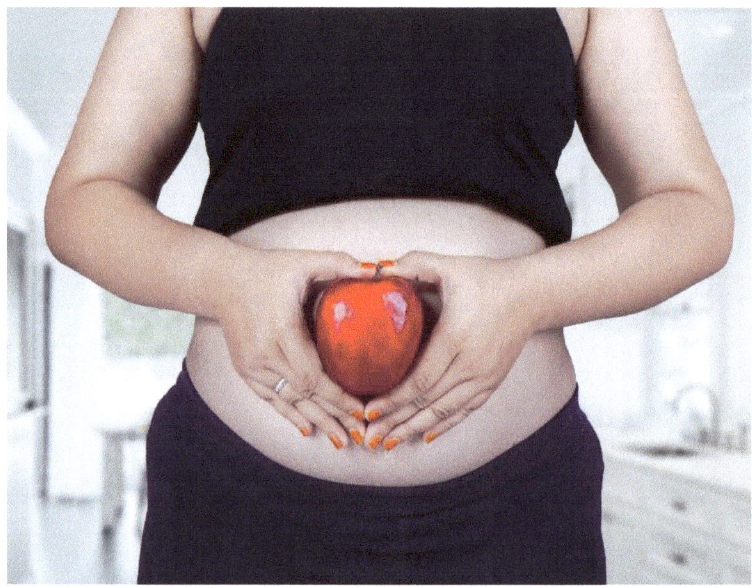

Apples are a great source of dietary fiber, with one medium apple containing about 4 grams of fiber. Fiber is important for digestion because it helps move food through your digestive tract and adds bulk to your stool, making it easier to pass. This can help prevent constipation and keep your digestive system running smoothly.

But that's not all – the fiber in apples also acts as a prebiotic, feeding the good bacteria in your gut. This can help promote a healthy balance of gut bacteria, which is important for digestion and overall health.

In addition to fiber, apples contain compounds called polyphenols, which have been shown to have anti-inflammatory effects in the gut. This can help reduce inflammation and irritation in your digestive system, reducing the risk of conditions like irritable bowel syndrome (IBS) and inflammatory bowel disease (IBD).

So, by eating apples, you're not only enjoying a delicious snack but also giving your tummy the fiber and nutrients it needs to stay healthy and happy. Next time you're feeling hungry, reach for an apple and give your digestive system a boost!

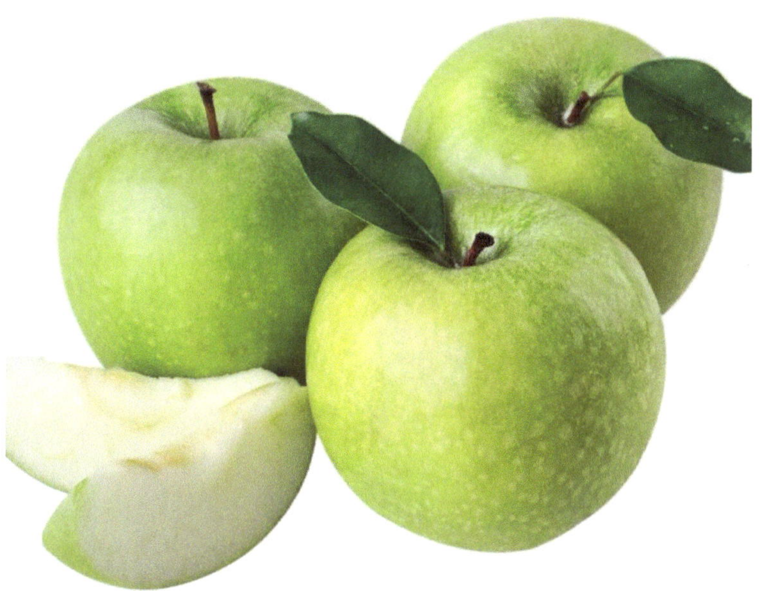

Chapter 6: An Apple for Your Teeth

Your smile is one of your most important features, and keeping your teeth healthy is key to maintaining a bright smile. In this chapter, we'll explore how apples can help keep your teeth healthy and your smile bright.

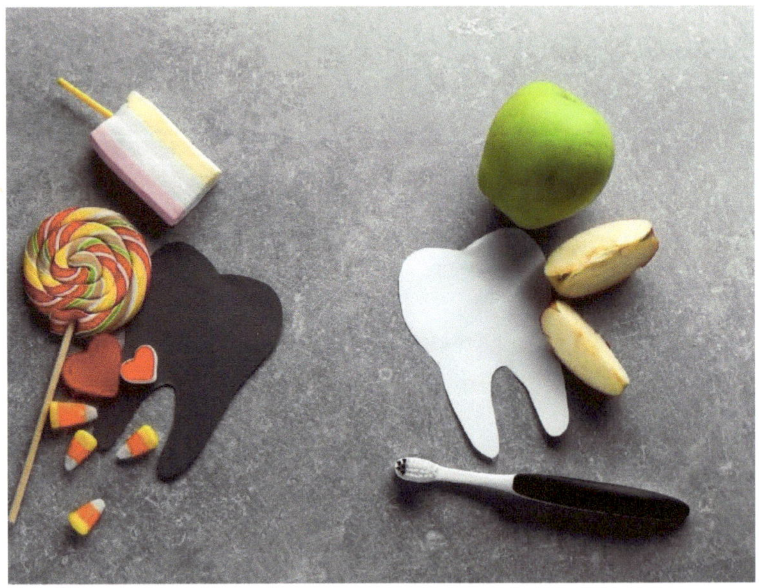

Apples contain natural acids, such as malic acid, which can help clean your teeth and remove stains. These acids stimulate the production of saliva, which is your mouth's natural defense against tooth decay. Saliva helps wash away food particles and neutralize acids produced by bacteria in your mouth, reducing the risk of cavities.

In addition to cleaning your teeth, the natural fibers in apples can also help scrub away plaque and debris, further reducing the risk of cavities and gum disease. Chewing apples can also help strengthen your gums, which are important for holding your teeth in place.

Not only do apples help keep your teeth clean, but they can also freshen your breath. The acids in apples help kill bacteria in your mouth that can cause bad breath, leaving your mouth feeling clean and refreshed.

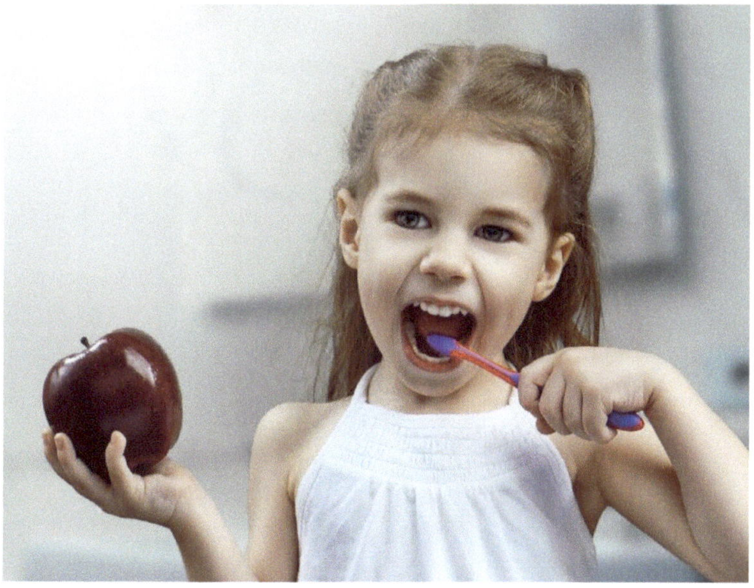

So, by eating apples, you're not only enjoying a delicious snack but also helping to keep your teeth healthy and your smile bright. Next time you're craving something sweet, reach for an apple and give your teeth some extra love!

Chapter 7: An Apple for Your Skin

Your skin is your body's largest organ and plays a vital role in protecting you from the outside world. It's important to take care of your skin to keep it looking healthy and youthful. In this chapter, we'll explore how apples can help keep your skin glowing and youthful.

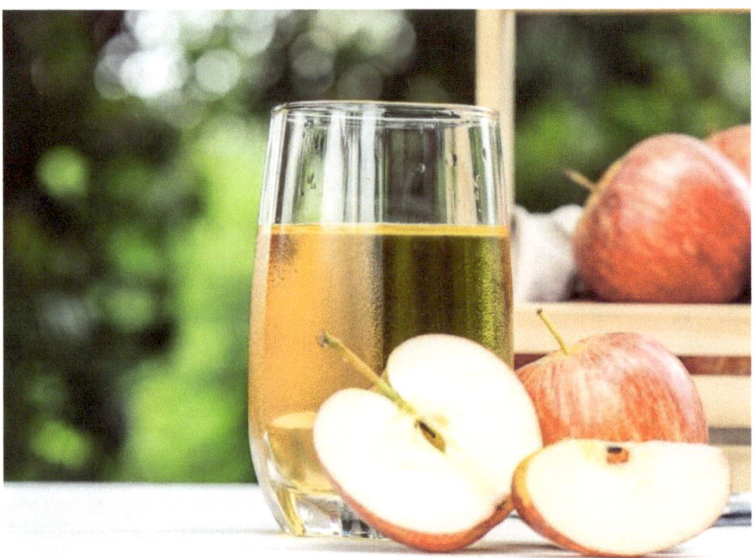

Apples are rich in vitamins and antioxidants that are beneficial for your skin. One of the key vitamins in apples is vitamin C, which is essential for the production of collagen, a protein that helps keep your skin firm and supple. Vitamin C also has antioxidant properties, which can help protect your skin from damage caused by free radicals, such as pollution and UV rays.

In addition to vitamin C, apples also contain other antioxidants, such as flavonoids and polyphenols, which have been shown to have anti-inflammatory and anti-aging effects on the skin. These antioxidants help reduce inflammation, prevent damage to skin cells, and promote skin repair, keeping your skin looking youthful and healthy.

Apples also contain a compound called quercetin, which has been shown to protect against UVB radiation, a type of radiation that can damage your skin and lead to premature aging. By eating apples, you can help protect your skin from the harmful effects of the sun and keep it looking its best.

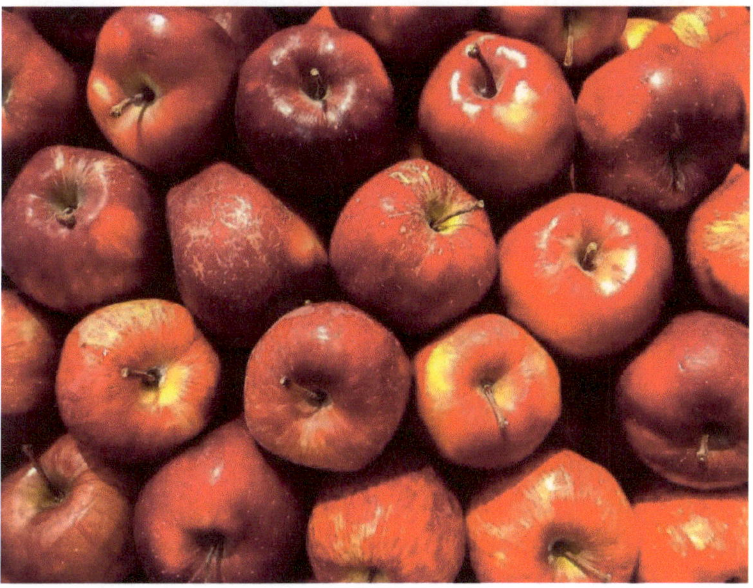

So, the next time you're looking for a snack, reach for an apple! Not only will it satisfy your taste buds, but it will also help keep your skin glowing and youthful.

Chapter 8: An Apple for Your Mood

Feeling down or stressed? Apples might just be the pick-me-up you need! In this chapter, we'll explore how apples can boost your mood and make you feel happy.

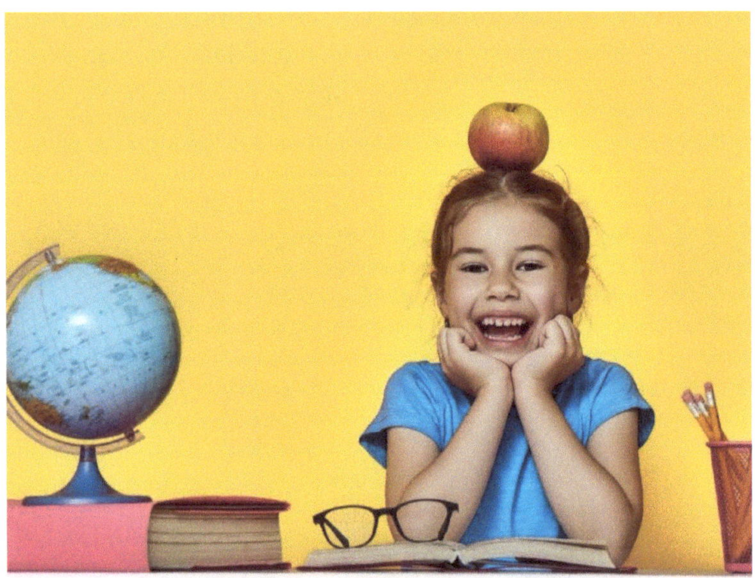

Apples contain several nutrients that are known to have mood-boosting effects. One of these nutrients is vitamin C, which has been shown to reduce stress and anxiety levels. Vitamin C helps regulate the production of cortisol, a hormone that is released in response to stress. By eating apples, you can help keep your cortisol levels in check and reduce feelings of stress and anxiety.

In addition to vitamin C, apples also contain antioxidants, such as quercetin, which have been shown to have anti-anxiety effects. Quercetin helps regulate the levels of neurotransmitters in the brain, such as serotonin and dopamine, which play a key role in mood regulation. By eating apples, you can help increase the production of these "feel-good" neurotransmitters, leaving you feeling calm and content.

Furthermore, the natural sugars in apples can provide a quick energy boost, which can help improve your mood and increase your overall sense of well-being. Unlike refined sugars, which can cause energy crashes, the sugars in apples are released slowly into the bloodstream, providing a steady source of energy without the crash.

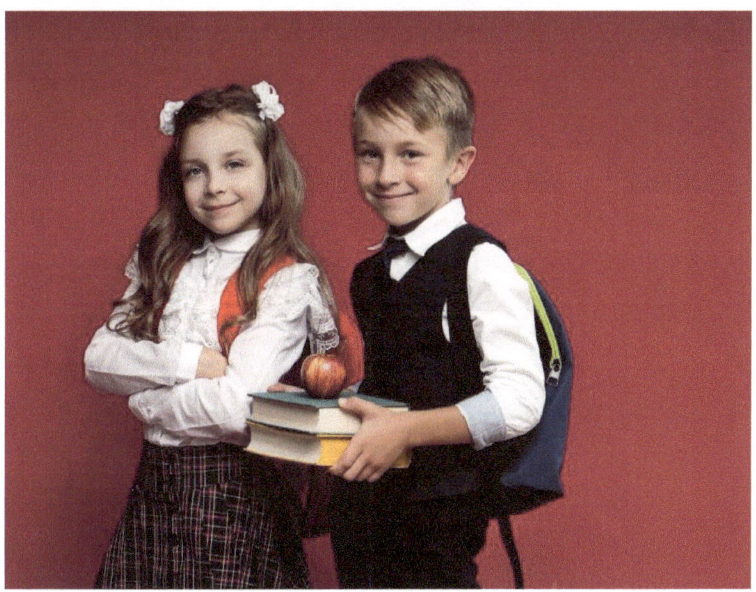

So, the next time you're feeling blue, reach for an apple! Not only will it satisfy your sweet tooth, but it will also help boost your mood and leave you feeling happy and content.

Conclusion:

Congratulations, young readers, you are now apple experts! Throughout this book, we've explored the many ways that apples can benefit your health and happiness. From boosting your immune system to keeping your heart healthy, apples are truly a superfood.

By adding apples to your diet, you can enjoy a wide range of benefits, including improved digestion, better skin health, and even a brighter smile. Whether you prefer them crunchy and sweet or soft and tart, there's no denying that apples are a delicious and nutritious snack.

So, the next time you're looking for a healthy snack, reach for an apple! Take a moment to savor its crisp texture and sweet flavor, knowing that you're giving your body a dose of vitamins, minerals, and antioxidants that will keep you feeling great.

Remember, an apple a day really can keep the doctor away! So, grab an apple, take a bite, and enjoy all the goodness it has to offer!

About the author Binish Shah

Binish Shah Expertise in sales management extends globally, where she crafts strategic approaches for various international companies. Her role involves devising tailored strategies for companies traversing the globe, leveraging her extensive sales experience and understanding of diverse markets.

Beyond her professional prowess, Binish Shah passion for personal development shines. She embraces mindfulness, honing its practical applications for enhanced focus and mental well-being. Her journey includes conquering stage fright, mastering public speaking, and fostering personal growth.

Financially astute, Binish Shah adeptly manages personal finances, drawing on her understanding of influence and persuasion across both professional and personal spheres.

Despite a busy schedule, maintaining a healthy lifestyle remains paramount to Binish Shah. She not only creates nutritious meals swiftly but also explores meditation practices for inner tranquility.

Emphasizing healthy relationships through effective communication and boundaries, Binish Shah values continual self-reflection and personal growth.

Networking stands as a cornerstone for her career advancement. She refines time management skills to maximize productivity and attain her objectives.

Her grasp of investment fundamentals enables informed financial decisions. To maintain equilibrium, Binish Shah delves into stress reduction techniques like mindfulness, yoga, and meditation, fostering a balanced mindset.

Yours Sincerely

Binish Shah

Description of the book:

"The Amazing Apple: A Fun Guide to the Benefits of Apples" is an engaging and educational book aimed at 5 to 12-year-olds. Through colorful illustrations and easy-to-understand language, this book explores the many ways that apples can benefit health and well-being.

Readers will discover how apples can boost the immune system, support healthy growth, and keep various body parts, such as the heart, brain, and skin, in top condition. Each chapter delves into a different aspect of apple benefits, such as digestion, dental health, and mood enhancement, making learning about nutrition both fun and informative.

By the end of the book, young readers will become apple experts, understanding the importance of incorporating this nutritious fruit into their daily diet. "The Amazing Apple" encourages children to grab an apple, take a bite, and enjoy all the goodness it has to offer!

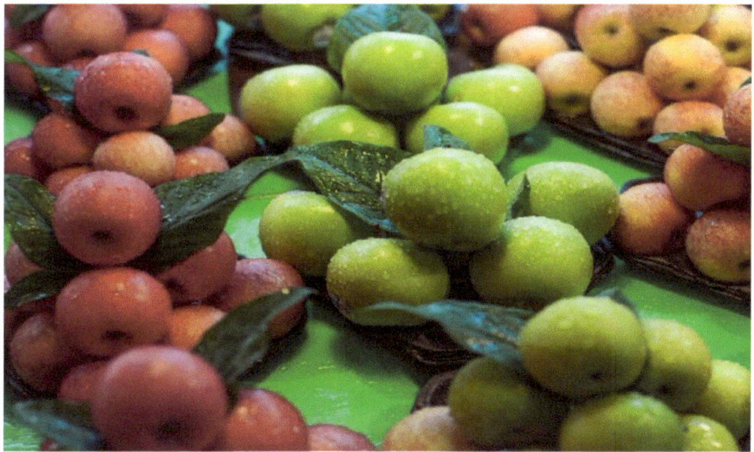

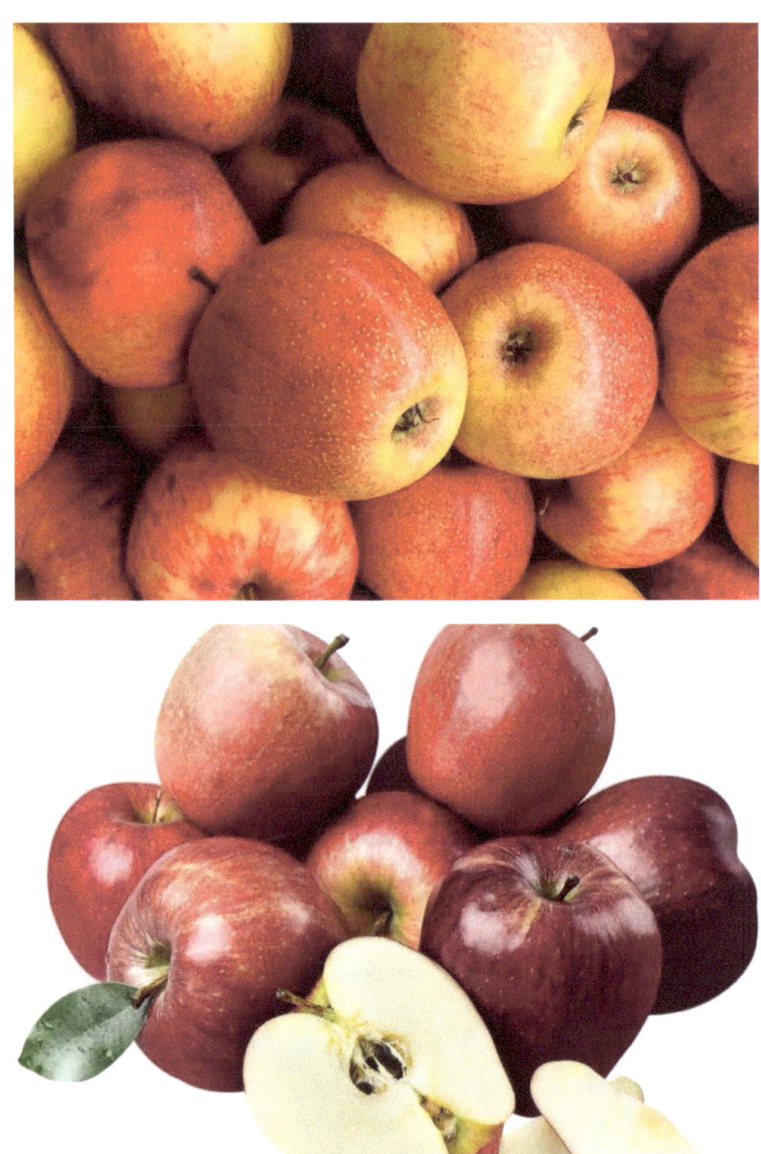

www.ingramcontent.com/pod-product-compliance
Lightning Source LLC
Chambersburg PA
CBHW040321240726

48664CB00006B/1584